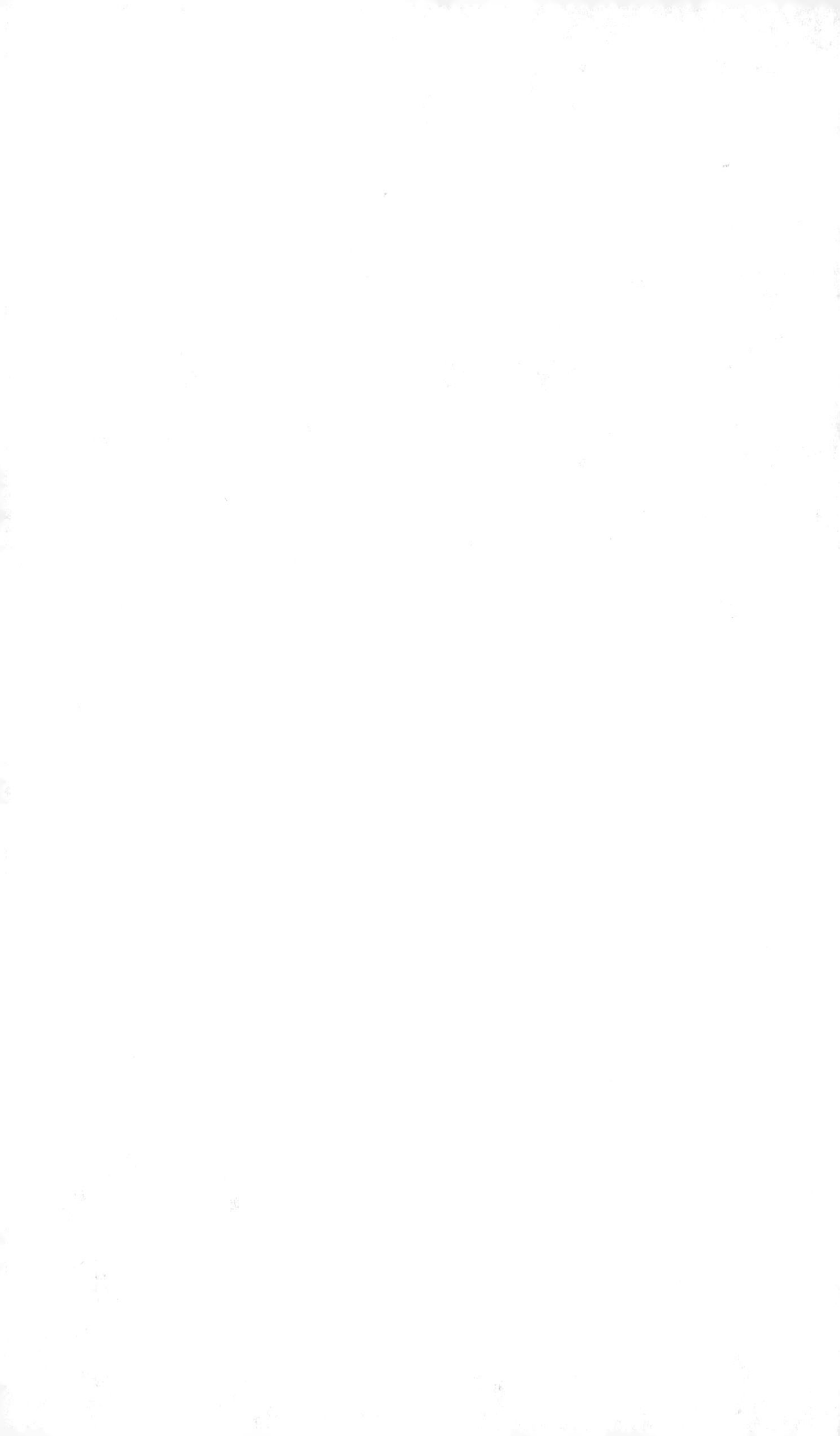

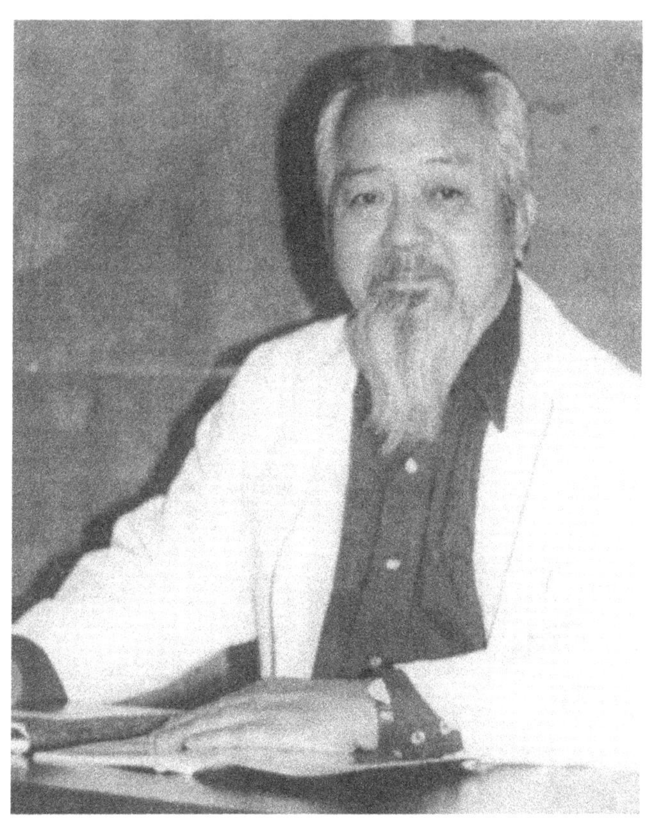

MIKOTO MASAHILO NAKAZONO

Founder of the Universal Institute (India 1955), the Kan Nagara Institute (Paris, France 1962), the Kototama Institute (Santa Fe, New Mexico 1978), and Inochi Resources, Inc. (Santa Fe, New Mexico 1985).

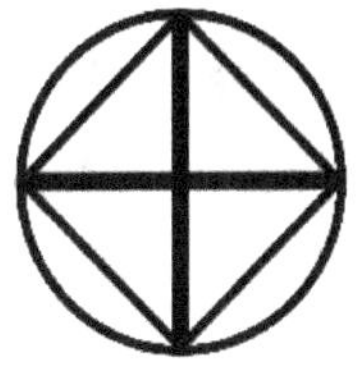

THE REAL SENSE OF NATURAL THERAPY

MIKOTO MASAHILO NAKAZONO

THE REAL SENSE OF NATURAL THERAPY

MIKOTO M. NAKAZONO

Published by Kototama Books
www.kototamabooks.com

ISBN-13: 978-0-9716674-3-3
ISBN-10: 0-9716674-3-8

Originally edited by Sarai Saporta, 1992.
Printed by Piñon Fast Print, Santa Fe, New Mexico, 2001.
Second printing: 2005.
Third Printing: Kindle Direct Publishing, 2023.

TABLE OF CONTENTS

FOREWORD

The original version of "The Real Sense of Natural Therapy" was written as a newsletter when the author first came to Santa Fe and realized how little informed the public was about natural therapy as an alternative to scientific treatment methods. This included only the first part of the book presented here. Later on he added the second part, to inform the New Mexico legislature when they were considering passing a bill to legalize acupuncture. With his leadership, the bill was passed. New Mexico was the first state in the union to introduce such a bill (the author's first attempt) but it took a few more years to have it accepted. The rest of this book is excerpts taken from the textbook of the Kototama Institute, directed toward the serious lay public who wish to have a broader and deeper understanding about health and healing and ultimately what it means to be a human being.

INTRODUCTION

This therapy is based on the life principle of Kototama Futomani. By this medical work, we are attempting to demonstrate that this principle is the final truth.

I have been a practitioner of oriental medicine for the past fifty years. Oriental medicine is one name but there are many different methods and groups of specialization within the same broad heading. These groups have their advantages and disadvantages but they have no fundamental general principle of the source of human disease. Western medicine is the same.

When I arrived at this life principle, I began to re-study oriental medicine, comparing it to the life principle. Gradually I began to understand that the medical principles based on the life principle were symbolically hidden in the *Yellow Emperor's Classic of Internal Medicine,* the *Nei-Ching,* our religious doctrines, cultural mythologies, etc. The content of the life principle was hinted at and all the ancient documents were based upon these hints. These documents of principles and theories were transmitted generation to generation and are the basis of today's oriental medicine.

Present human beings must try to understand the true meaning of our ancestors' thoughts and teachings. First we must renounce our present knowledge and return "as a new born baby", our minds a blank piece of paper, and begin to search for the real source of ourselves – our substance.

The original way of civilization was based on the view of the life dimension's world; their medical therapies were the same. However, after the life principle was hidden in symbolic hints, these hints became the foundation of today's "oriental medicine". Today, oriental medicine and oriental civilization have no way to grasp the content of the substance. They have lost it.

For the past twenty years I have searched and practiced so as to grasp the life principle. The present situation of civilization has to be based on this principle. I founded this life therapy with the intention of proving the Way of Truth.

Masahilo M. Nakazono
Santa Fe, N.M. 1985

THE REAL SENSE OF NATURAL THERAPY

Healing can never be perfected as long as the treatment is confined to the maintenance of our physical existence. We need to realize the total relationship of human beings to the plants, earth, water, heat and air, as well as to the earth and heaven. Until that time comes, humanity will continue to fear sickness and death.

When aspirin was first discovered, it was thought that this would be the end of colds. Penicillin, antibiotics, steroids and other powerful new drugs have since helped some lives, yet the number of sick people is on the increase. It seems the more new drugs are discovered, the more new illnesses emerge which cannot be cured by them. We are all well aware of this situation, particularly those in the health care community. Doctors who honestly confront their responsibility must suffer because of it. It is the most painful experience for a doctor to see a patient he or she cannot help. Yet even with this sense of sadness, people all over the world die every day – babies, young people and the aged. Why does this happen when we have so many new and improved therapies today?

Scientific research has almost completed its understanding of the body's physical nature, but still sickness cannot be cured. Why? We must wake up and discover the answer to this question. Many people have already touched on this point, but no one has yet found the answer.

As a student of natural therapy, I am particularly interested in studying the world of the life will. The principle of the life will was found and perfected by our ancient forebears but it has entirely been forgotten. This loss saddens me, so that whenever I can, I try to explain it to others through my writing and speaking. I am always attempting to contact other real students of the truth.

In any discussion of natural therapy, we must also speak about modern therapy and find the basic premise behind each of these disciplines. We must discover the relationship between the spiritual civilization of ten thousand years ago, and today's material civilization which began about four thousand years ago. Until four thousand years ago, there were no nations – there were no borders. As was written in the Bible, the whole world spoke one language – the one Word – and that was the peaceful and perfect era of the Garden of Eden. We think of this period as something of a myth, a fable which no one takes seriously. Nevertheless, it did exist. The destruction of the Tower of Babel was the destruction of the one language of human beings which marks the beginning of the separation inherent in the material civilization.

The biblical symbolism conceals the one principle which had been the basis of the spiritual civilization. From the beginning of the material civilization, all that had been a unified whole began to be separated, moving further and further away from this one principle. This current of civilization has continued into our present era. Medicine, in the context of civilization, is obliged to evolve along the same lines, i.e., to separate from the principle of the first civilization. You may think ancient history has no relationship to medical therapies, but, until this fact is understood, we will not find a solution to today's difficulties.

The first civilization was based on the principle of the totality of life. The second civilization is based on the scientific study of each part of the objective limited world – the world of limited phenomena. It studies that which we can see and grasp with the physical senses. In studying the object, we lose the subject and human beings become another object in the phenomenal world. We believe the subject can be found by starting with a scientific study of the object, but it can never be found in that direction. The subject does not come after the object. Until our search can take a different turn, we will always search in vain.

In studying the objective world, we begin by dissecting it more and more minutely, destroying the object's form, sacrificing the integrity of the whole for its parts. Who can say how much life has been sacrificed to develop today's modern medicine? Without sacrificing the form, the scientific civilization could not have been completed. We can clearly see that this way of destruction – the dissection of life – belongs to the same current of separation which divides all areas of civilization into separate languages, countries and religions. As it intensifies, more and more separate theories will emerge. The great leaders of the first civilization prophesied that this would occur and left us many descriptions of our age in seemingly mythological stories.

In the current of this age, it is impossible for medical work, all by itself, to hold on to the truth; it naturally reflects its time. To perfect any therapy, to rebuild a perfect society, to turn away from this complex mental haze, we must re-discover the spiritual principle – the ancient truth of our ancestors. There is no other way.

The human being is a materialization from the void – from the world of nothing. Humans are the manifestation of the one life will of the universe which separates into individual human life forms. This is the truth of human existence. That human beings are distinct from animals and plants is also a truth, but all formed life emerges from the void in this way. It is the human ego which asserts that we alone are true and real, and can therefore sacrifice all other forms of the same truth and reality. To destroy any form of natural life is equivalent to the destruction of the truth. This we must recognize. If the human body's life was separate from all other existence, there would be a different life principle. However, it is not separate. Our existence is directly related to all others. Even the smallest virus cannot be separated from this principle of life.

Destroying any kind of life form, for any reason, goes directly against the law of universal existence and must not be continued.

When, using intellectual knowledge, we artificially cause the breaking up of one kind of life form, it seems that it has been completely destroyed. While the actual structure seen with the physical eye has been lost, the source of that form's life will can never die. Actually, it has just been separated into smaller and smaller forms. These smaller forms continue to unite with other life forms, and eventually, a new virus emerges to again plague humanity. We do not realize that we alone created this new virus by destroying its predecessor. It is folly to say we have killed some kind of life. The life will is the life of the universe itself, manifesting phenomena as separate and different forms of itself. Breaking up one phenomenal form, the life will returns to the source or incorporates with other life forms. We must perfectly realize this.

When we kill or break up a virus with drugs, the life will of the virus either returns to the universal source, or reincorporates into the human system as a different, smaller form, or is eliminated from the body and incorporates itself into plants, animals, or other life forms. Only its form has been altered; the virus can never truly be killed. Simultaneously, with the use of strong drugs, the human body has also received a shock. We think that killing the virus with strong drugs does not cause any harmful effects to the body, but this is not true. Unicellular forms are far more adaptive than the human constitution.

Physical life is the embodiment of the motive vibration of the universe. There are stronger and weaker forms of life energy and a stronger force will change a weaker one. When modern drug therapy shocks the body's system, the form of the body's cells is changed. If cigarettes or very strong food can be seen as the cause of cancer, we must be more judicious in our use of powerful drugs. We cannot see how their vibrations influence the body's constitution, altering and reforming it. In the near future, no doubt a drug will be discovered that can "cure" cancer. At that moment, we humans will be the recipients of some new, as yet unknown, difficulties such as new disease-causing viruses – the result of the breaking up of the cancer virus.

Using such things as vitamins can give some added strength to a particular part of the body, but it is often too one-sided. The parts of the body function in two ways, positive and negative. Giving too much energy to one side is detrimental to the other. One side wins, one side loses and the exhaustion of the nervous system is the result. Even if both positive and negative aspects are carefully taken into consideration, it is very difficult to know how to balance them correctly when introducing any special substances into the body. Each positive-negative system has its own uniquely fluctuating balance.

To put it briefly, acupuncture, or rather, life therapy, is based on the flow of the life will's energy current through twelve main channels (or meridians) of the body. Ten of these meridians correspond to vital organs and there are special points on each of these meridians which are most effective for treatment. Sickness can be said to result from an unbalanced circulation of energy throughout the body.

When balance is re-established, the flow of energy is normal and the sickness disappears. All organs are intimately related; the imbalance of one directly affects the others.

Modern medicine cannot see that the cause of a patient's kidney infection may not be due directly to the kidneys but to the imbalance of the lung or some other organ whose symptoms have not yet appeared. A person prone to kidney infections may be receiving medication for them, but continues to have kidney infections for a number of years. Years later, when another organ fails, modern medicine will not see that this failing organ was the cause of the earlier kidney problems. Life therapy, by a system of reading the pulses of each organ, searches for the real cause of the illness. While treating the symptoms of disease, it also treats its source.

I am not saying that modern medicine is of no use. The question is, how to use it? Usually, modern medicine over stimulates the human system, giving it too much energy. What is most important, the strength or quantity of dosage? In order to judge this correctly, we must first understand the relationship of the body's life to universal life. Oriental medicine is based on this life principle and has treated human sickness from this point of view from very ancient times.

Western medicine has nearly completed its investigation of the actual human body. Oriental medicine knows little about this, but it does have the knowledge of thousands of years of relationship to the life principle. Originally this principle forbade the killing of any kind of life since all forms of existence have equal claim to life in the limited world. They are all manifestations of the one universal source. Mental illness is the result of our exclusive human ego which denies the universal law. This kind of egoism can destroy whatever enters its limited space. If we remember this seriously, such a notion can be clearly seen as mistaken. Whoever opposes the law of the universe is obliged to suffer the repercussions of his actions.

This sense is completely different from that of today's society. As I explained, it comes from the direction of today's modern current, i.e., separation. "I am separate so how can my actions affect the universe?" Once the universal law is violated however, there is no escaping the consequences. Such important matters have been forgotten by uncaring human beings. Their attitude finally results in the mutual killing of other humans without feelings of remorse – deadening any inner sense of pain that would normally flow from such an action.

This attitude is the result of our intelligence and our physical sense of the body. Intelligence means the accumulation of past experience. With only these two dimensions of human capacity, we cannot grasp the source of our life. We must begin to use the other three dimensions of our existence. This subject will not be discussed here but interested readers may refer to my book, "Inochi, the Book of Life." Human capacity separates into five dimensions and human therapy cannot be perfected until we have grasped all of these dimensions.

Oriental practitioners of natural therapy are divided into three categories: Jio – Yi, the supreme doctor; Chiu – Yi, the average doctor; and Ka – Yi. The last category, Ka –

Yi, treats the physical sicknesses of the human body. The middle category, Chiu – Yi, treats sickness before it manifests, i.e., preventive therapy. The highest category, Jio – Yi, treats the sickness of society – the sickness of the collective human mind, also as preventive therapy.

Most people are not aware of the source of their desires, much less do they even attempt to study them. Their goal is simply to immediately satisfy the desires of the moment, and then to increase the means of satisfying them more fully. The point of view from this dimension creates a greed for food, sex, clothes, and for accumulating more money and property. Despite the fact that we have five dimensions, when our main desire is to satisfy physical need, our life will seems to manifest only in that one dimension. It would be better if physical satisfaction were kept to a minimum. When, however, we seek blindly to satisfy only the physical dimension, not only is greed endless, but habits are created which have an endless energy of their own.

For example, when a greedy habit in relation to food is established, the automatic result is physical sickness. For that reason, Oriental natural therapy says that sickness begins with the mouth. Diet treatment is based upon this premise. Professor Ohsawa's macrobiotics, using the yin-yang/negative-positive principle based on a concept in the "I-Ching", is a well-known method of diet in Europe and America. This principle, however, does not go far enough in considering the differences of climate and geography on the individual, nor the individual's specific weaknesses and needs.

There are many other diet methods and while they are all different, they all recommend the eating of natural foods. All these different methods are another example of the current of separation in our civilization. They are all based on the respective founder's personal and separate experience and are a reflection of each one's native climate, geography, and time. Here again, the loss of the original life principle is clearly evident, yet each one of these different methods attracts a certain following. Regardless of the differences in time, climate and upbringing, people blindly follow systems they cannot understand. Only the principle they hold in common can be true, that of eating natural foods.

What is the relationship of the earth to the human body? Our planet is a combination of fire (heat), water, earth, plant and animal life. These five levels of life are very clearly divided but they are also interrelated. For example, earth, water and heat give life to the plant world. Likewise, plants give life to animals and there are animals who subsist on the meat of other animals which were plant eaters. This forms a direct link between the animal and plant worlds, the order being fixed and unchanging. Within this order of universal life, the human body must be placed in a harmonious position. This principle of life, however, is not included in today's Asiatic diet methods.

Further influences are the dimensions of air, sun, moon, stars and infinity. The physical life of the human body manifests from the world of infinity first and undergoes transformations from these ordered influences. Simultaneously, the body is also influenced by the categories previously mentioned which culminate in plants and animals. This is the way the human body is produced.

Our human body exists within such a relationship and depends on the orderly flow of all these other dimensions. If we search deeply for the origins of our body's life, we can see this order of the universe and our body's relationship to it; the journey of these formative influences and transformations can be recognized. This profound recognition is the intelligence of our life will – the human seed. This kind of intelligence can also be the future continuation of this process of infinite development. Once we use this intelligence, the complete order of our body's mechanism can be discovered. Thus an instantaneous synchronization can occur between oncoming influences and our life will.

The life will creates the body and sustains its life. If the goal of education in a society were the awakening of this original faculty, there would no longer be a need for that special occupation of "doctor", nor even for the use of therapy in the future. This may sound extreme, but it is true. It may cause anger in some, but the origin of medicine is the expression of that part of the life will which protects and maintains our natural human life. The weakest life is nurtured in the same way. Medical therapies were originally a specialization created by this divine love and morality of the highest order. If this original principle of therapy is remembered, my tone will be completely understood.

Professor Ohsawa, the founder of macrobiotics, always said that sick people are the same as criminals and should be given no respect. We have our original human faculty and can see and know all of this ourselves. We are unable to use our total capacity, however, and when we are sick it means we have violated the universal law. When we do not exercise this faculty, it is the same as not wanting to breathe air, or avoiding the sunlight.

Since the loss of the principle of life we humans recognize only two dimensions: the physical senses and the intelligence of the intellect; and we have created a civilization based on these two alone.

The basic principles of oriental natural therapy were also gradually lost. Today, it is a school course system and there is no longer any study of the life will principle. The result is only an intellectual learning of healing techniques; the life behind them is not understood. It is for this reason that, no matter how much either modern medicine or the points of acupuncture are studied, sickness cannot always be cured. For example, the Saninko point on the spleen meridian greatly affects the ovaries. If you treat this point over a period of time, you may have excellent results. Yet, at other times, there may be no response, or the condition may even get worse. All of these results can occur with the same patient, treated to the same degree.

At different times of the year, or even of the day, a patient's reactions will vary greatly – according to the weather, the digestion of food, and many other reasons. We should not have to learn from others how to have this kind of sensitivity. If natural therapy forgets about the relationship between the body and these other factors, concentrating only on technique, there is little difference between it and modern medicine.

Natural therapy treatment, through handwork, needles, moxa, herbs and diet has as its objective the balance of the flow of life energy. It gives energy to those parts of the body that need it and removes it from those that are over-energized. This unblocks the energy and allows it to circulate freely. This balancing restores the natural condition of the body's vibration, putting it back into harmony with the universal vibration. Diet, for example, influences the digestion and conversion of food which gives the body its energy so that it can function harmoniously and with the internal and external universal vibrations. A good diet thus creates a good body vibration which can more readily adapt to the changing vibrations of the universe.

Modern medicine has exactly the same objective but it is based on the idea of fighting with the illness. This attitude is unacceptable to the real sense of natural therapy because the cutting off or breaking up of any kind of life form is contrary to the natural law of the universe. When a mistake is made we must accept the judgement of the universe. Those consequences descend upon both doctor and patient alike, not on one side alone. When our society returns to the study of life, everyone will understand this. A concentrated study of the methods and techniques of treatment which forgets the study of life is not the way. Should this attitude continue, competition between human and other life forms will never cease. That is why we must try to grasp the real principle of the source of our life.

Although natural therapy, reflecting the trend of today, has lost its ability to use the one life principle, it has nevertheless retained a symbolic explanation of the source of our life within its treatment and theory. It must be rediscovered and grasped and a cooperative relationship with modern medicine established. An attempt must be made to develop a therapeutic method that is perfect. For one hundred years, modern medicine has held sway over human society, but it should not try to repress the emergence of natural therapy now. Modern medicine needs this principle. Oriental natural therapy has the historical experience of many thousands of years and modern therapy can study many things gleaned from this experience. This much should be apparent: medical therapy is not the property of a few. It belongs to all human beings and everyone should seriously work together for its perfection. As long as we follow the current of separation we will not do this, or any other work, for humanity.

I have tried in this brief article to explain something of the total aspect of therapy in the world and how it must be related to all other parts of civilization. I have not delved into treatment methods very much because there are other books readily available on the subject. I must add that it is always difficult to explain in any book the real sense of natural therapy, and, as to methods of treatment, nothing can be truly conveyed in words.

THE DIFFERENCE BETWEEN NATURAL AND MODERN THERAPY

Natural therapy, the therapy of life, first became known to our ancient ancestors many thousands of years ago. They were able to use their inner eye to see the activity of the universe and the order in which life is made manifest. They could see the source of human life, with all its capacity, and could understand the body's sickness from this cosmic point of view.

This method of healing seeks the cause of illness in the unbalanced circulation of energy which appears as abnormal symptoms of the body. Its objective is to normalize the currents of life energy by bringing them into balance again. It deals with energy on an a priori level, before its materialization as a physical body.

Modern medicine is concerned with the elements of the physical body after it has been formed. It deals with that dimension of human life after the sperm and egg have combined, generating more cells and their growth into specialized functions such as organs, bones, skin, etc. When some part of the body acts abnormally, the dysfunction itself is called a disease and given a name. The doctor seeks to heal a particular part of the body, where the abnormal condition is. This is the research and technique of a posteriori therapy.

Natural therapy and modern therapy stand on two different dimensions of life. From two such diverse perspectives, it would necessarily follow that the methods of diagnosis and treatment would be entirely different.

Ultimately, to understand what natural therapy is, one must know what a human being is. One must first be clear about the source of human physical life – its activity and capabilities. In the same breath, one has to be talking about the life of the universe, in both its finite and infinite activity. It is this part of life that science does not include. For science, this dimension's world is unclear.

To give a brief explanation of natural therapy is close to impossible. Nevertheless, I will try to give a simplified version for those who are interested in studying this method, and for the general public who would like some basic knowledge of the subject.

The principles of natural therapy are a legacy from many thousands of years ago. What these ancient people could grasp was that the total action of the life of the universe and that of human life have one source.

It was with this understanding that the human beings of ancient times created a civilization. All over the world, that time has been preserved in symbolic form through myths, prophecies, philosophies, religions, etc. The original principles of natural therapy, as found in the old documents, are a part of this legacy. They are the most important documents to guide modern civilization back to the way of truth.

In the ancient documents, the manner and terminology of the text are far from scientific, so a literal translation would be incomprehensible to the modern mind. To explain their contents, therefore, I shall borrow from the language of science, in order to translate their meaning.

All universal life and its physical manifestation are from one source. Its activity constantly changes, but it can never be made less; the sum total of life energy remains permanently unchanged.

Universal activity is based on the one greatest center of the universe which scientifically has not yet been understood. Within it is a void; pure, no-thing. It naturally attracts elements from outside, which, being heavier, fall into the void. The void is concentrating, or gravity power. This closing action continues until it reaches a critical point and then begins pushing the elements back out, in the expanding direction.

Thus the center acts in two opposite ways, concentrating and expanding. In ancient China, the action of expansion was given the symbolic name of Yang and concentration was called Yin.

From the greatest center, the life energy of the universe has two modes of expansion: the total universe expands and at the same time, at the extremes of expansion, it also separates. The time and space for these two kinds of expansion occur in the world of infinity. This cannot be grasped from the dimension of the human, physical eye.

When energy cannot expand any further, either as a totality or in its separated parts, it turns back in the direction of concentration, going back into the greatest center. This also happens in two modes: the force of the total universe concentrates and each separated part individually concentrates, creating small whirlpools of energy.

It is in this moment of concentration that the beginning of the finite world is created: particles, molecules, atoms, etc. These combine to create the next level of formed existence. They keep joining, building larger and larger forms. Life energy continues to create the different dimensions of space this way, from smaller to larger.

This action of concentrating and joining creates four separate dimensions of universal energy. Science has already grasped that energy has four dimensions (Dr. Murray Gell-Mann). Their activity, when in the concentrating direction, finally creates the finite world, the dimensions that are perceivable with the physical senses.

The total finite world keeps concentrating, moving step by step, in time, closer to the greatest center. All form finally disappears, swallowed into the void of the greatest center. This means all form returns to the source energy where it changes and again takes the expanding direction.

Today science has conceptualized a black hole theory where each black hole controls a certain limited space in the universe in the center of a galaxy. A black hole (what I call a void center) is the end point of the concentration of the galactic system. In time, all the galaxy's physical elements will be swallowed by its black hole, including light, and from there will change to its expanding direction of energy. This is all within the space of that galactic system.

This action is of the same nature as the greatest center of the universe, as previously described. The difference is one of size. The greatest center's activity includes the total space of the universe and is perpetual. The black holes detected by science are limited to the bounds of each galaxy. Compared to our life span their activity seems permanent, but actually, they too have a limited life span.

The life energy of the total universe is based on this greatest center and is continuously expanding and concentrating from there. Automatically, these two waves of energy, spiraling in opposite directions, will meet and synchronize everywhere in the space of the universe.

At the moment and place of synchronization, these two opposite spiraling waves create whirlpools of life energy

– larger, smaller, stronger, weaker, etc. The whirlpool is the space in which all finite phenomena are created; it is the source of the space and time of all finite phenomena.

Each whirlpool's activity is of exactly the same nature as that of the greatest center. That is, each one has a void center and acts in two modes of expansion and two of concentration. The difference is that these a priori whirlpools are limited in time and space. The gravity power of each center determines the differences of age and spatial area: longer, shorter, larger, smaller, etc.

Each whirlpool will also grow in strength and enlarge its space just as a young life will grow up and reach maturity. At the height of its power, the center's strength will start to diminish. After collecting to its maximum, the whirlpool weakens and its power is absorbed by other, younger whirlpools nearby. These changes, from increase to decrease of a priori life activity, manifest the age of a posteriori life for all finite, physical phenomena.

The life energy of a whirlpool acts not only within its two modes of expansion and two modes of concentration, but also in five dimensions. This is the action of a priori life and it is the substance of the human being. It is the capacity of self.

From ancient times, natural therapy gave a symbolic name to this life activity (which divides into five dimensions). It called the five dimensions gogio – the five elements. For each dimension's energy, it used a symbolic name taken from nature: wood, fire, earth, metal, water.

A priori human life energy, then, separates into gogio – (mok, ka, do, gon, sui), spiraling within each whirlpool and sustaining thereby a certain limited space. It attracts the elements it needs from its immediate environment, concentrating and increasing itself, creating the material of the physical body, giving it life and capacity. When the life power of the five a priori elements is at its earlier stage of development, it creates smaller a posteriori forms such as sperm, eggs, primary cells, etc. As its power increases, by combining with other whirlpools it has attracted, the combined energy also creates a stronger physical body. That is how the human body grows to maturity. When it has developed to its fullest, the body strength begins to wane. Sickness refers to abnormal conditions of the physical constitution; that is, each person's abnormal mental or physical feelings. Modern therapy utilizes the scientific method to uncover the cause of such conditions by examining the body itself. The objective of treatment is to repair that part of the body which is dysfunctional. Natural therapy searches for the abnormal activity of the five a priori dimensions of life energy and adjusts their malsynchronization.

The methods of diagnosis and treatment of natural therapy deal with the currents of five dimensions of energy, or meridians. It finds which current and direction has lost balance, which current is out of synchronization with the others – which part of the body is out of harmony with the rest.

The four ways of diagnosis are: seeing, hearing, questioning and touching. Natural therapy then tries to normalize the circulation of life energy within the space of the body.

Natural therapy works exclusively to maintain a perfect condition of the circulation of the five a priori dimensions' energy in the space of the human body. It also tries to bring all physical life into harmony with the life of the universe, as one activity that follows the same rhythm, order and law.

The name of a disease as deduced by modern medicine can be of some help diagnostically. However, by capably following the correct procedures of traditional methods of diagnosis and treatment, it is not necessary to know the name of the disease; all types of disease will naturally be cured.

It is not the techniques of natural therapy that do the healing. It is the judgment of each person's life substance that heals the body it has created. Technique is solely for the manipulation of life energy currents. Modern medicine tries to heal a disease directly with the physical body. For natural therapy, the healer is the universal law; for modern therapy, it is the human being that is the healer of the disease.

Modern therapy has, of course, made great strides with its advanced methods of treatment and the use of drugs, more powerful than natural methods. However, its basic point of view limits itself to the boundaries of the physical system. It does not grasp the law of the a priori world.

With its powerful treatment techniques, modern therapy can successfully heal that part of the body which is diseased but it also destroys the other parts of the body. For natural therapy, it is forbidden to violate the law of life by breaking down the body's parts. Doctors and patients do not realize that this is in fact what they are doing.

In the foregoing, I have given only a very rough explanation of the differences in healing between natural and modern therapies. It was not meant as a criticism of modern methods. The two should be working together.

For the last few hundred years, the scientific method has searched exclusively in the physical realm. It has almost completely clarified the question of the human physical constitution. So many people, East and West, have given the energy of a lifetime to develop modern therapy. I give all of them my deepest respect and gratitude for their devotion.

My hope is that modern therapy can take one step further and research the a priori life world, which creates physical life. My hope and prayer is not for the benefit of the individual practitioner but for the perfection of the therapy of this civilization. My hope is also the hope of all humanity.

Natural therapy has the broadest concept of the universe. It requires a minimum of ten years' study in order to grasp this sense. After ten years, you may consider yourself a beginner; that is the traditional teaching from ancient times. When I reflect about my experience of the last fifty years, I can say this teaching is true; it is exactly like that.

Whoever wishes to search this way must get over their greed and ulterior motives – whatever ideas they have from their lower dimensions. Without talking too much, they must quietly go the straight road, working to perfect this human therapy. They must have a pure mind as a missionary, with strong confidence and courage.

If they cannot reach toward their higher dimensions' inner morality, then consciously or not, they destroy the truth. From the outset, they have no capacity as healers. People who continue the wrong way must know they are destroying the truth and that, sooner or later, they are obliged to suffer the punishment of the universal law, the law of God. They must finally destroy themselves.

The epoch of the material-scientific civilization is drawing to a close and the time is coming for all human beings to return to the way of truth and justice.

SELF – HEALTH

SOUND EXERCISE

The Kototama sounds in Futonorito order. Starting with **A**, read from right **A, I, E, O, U...TA, TI, TE...** and then **A, TA, KA, MA, HA, LA, NA, YA, SA, WA...I, TI, KI...**

WA	**SA**	**YA**	**NA**	**LA**	**HA**	**MA**	**KA**	**TA**	**A**
WI	**SI**	**YI**	**NI**	**LI**	**HI**	**MI**	**KI**	**TI**	**I**
WE	**SE**	**YE**	**NE**	**LE**	**HE**	**ME**	**KE**	**TE**	**E**
WO	**SO**	**YO**	**NO**	**LO**	**HO**	**MO**	**KO**	**TO**	**O**
WU	**SU**	**YU**	**NU**	**LU**	**HU**	**MU**	**KU**	**TU**	**U**

These sounds are the basic life rhythms at the bottom of human physical life. From ancient times, religions speak of the Word of God, and these are the contents of the Word. This exercise is for grasping the meaning of each sound rhythm, that is, one's own substance. The sounds are voiced using the entire body, as both a physical and spiritual purification exercise.

Each sound should be pronounced exactly, one at a time. It is helpful at first to practice with other, more experienced students.

Make each sound for as long as possible in one breath and with full voice.

A as in "ah" - the mouth is fully open, big and round.
I as in "we" - bite the teeth, opening the lips sideways.
E as in "way" - from the **I** position, open the teeth.
O as in "oh" - open mouth half-way, making it round.
U as in "who" - make the mouth small and round.

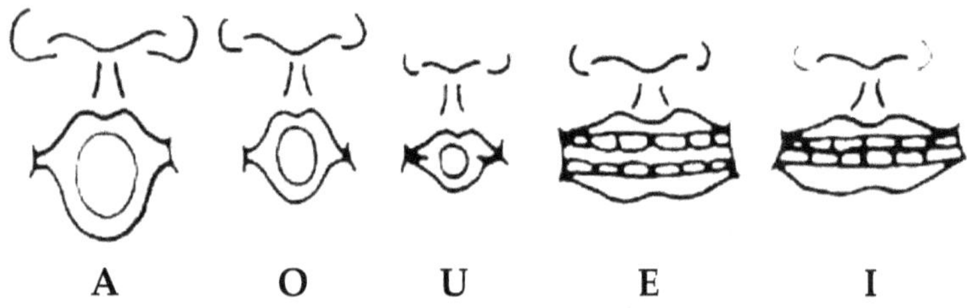

A O U E I

Do this exercise breathing deeply and with the deepest concentration of spirit. It may be done sitting or standing, but the body should be pulled up with a straight spine. Sound out from the tanden, located a few inches below the navel.

BREATHING THERAPY

a) Breathe quietly and slowly. At the end of each in breath, breathe in three more short breaths and then exhale slowly. At the end of each exhale, breathe out three short breaths.

b) After practicing awhile, try to lengthen the time of each direction of breathing, but be careful about your strength and capacity. This exercise should not be forced.

c) This exercise is best done in the morning but not in polluted air.

d) Exercise in a sitting, standing or lying down (on the back) position.

RUBBING THERAPY

a) Rub your hand all over your body. Wherever you feel a stiffness or pain, slightly press down on it for awhile.

b) Using a 100% cotton dry cloth or towel, rub the entire body until it has warmed up.

c) Dip a towel into cold water and ring it out. Rub it all over the body until the skin becomes red. Do not do this if you are catching cold or if you have a fever.

SHOWER THERAPY

a) Use alternating hot and cold showers, thirty seconds hot and thirty seconds cold, repeating two or three times. After becoming habituated, lengthen the time to one minute each. The last shower should be cold. During the shower, vigorously rub the body with a tawashi or towel until the skin radiates.

b) At first, hot and cold temperatures should not be too extreme. When feeling stronger, slowly widen the temperatures, a little colder and a little warmer. Later on you may start with cold, alternate with hot, finishing with cold.

c) This exercise trains the body physically and spiritually and improves its adaptive ability, to better synchronize with outside changes in temperature. It also helps blood circulation and strengthens the skin. In the beginning, do not force it too much and do not hurry along the way. It should be done according to the body's condition and strength and not more than twice a day.

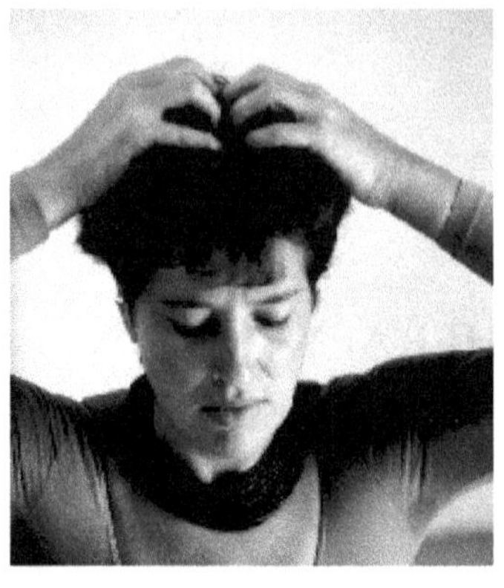

SELF-EXERCISE

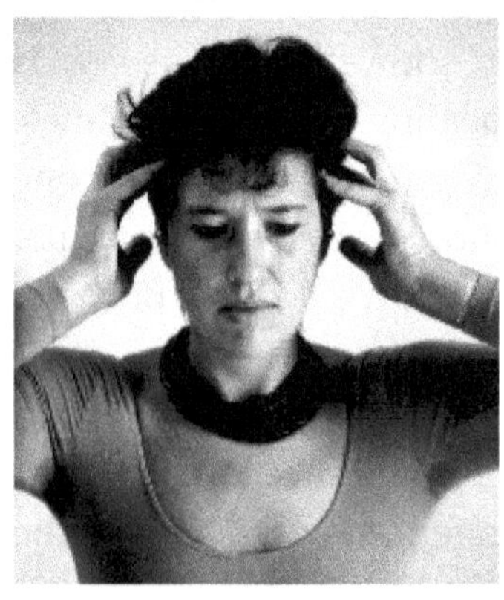

Head: Do shiatsu (pressure) on the head with your fingers, starting from the center line, and going down on the sides all around your head. Under the base of the skull, press up with the thumbs. Press everywhere on the face – eyes, ears, nose, under the jaw, the chin, the throat and all around the back of the neck. Wherever it feels sensitive, press a little more.

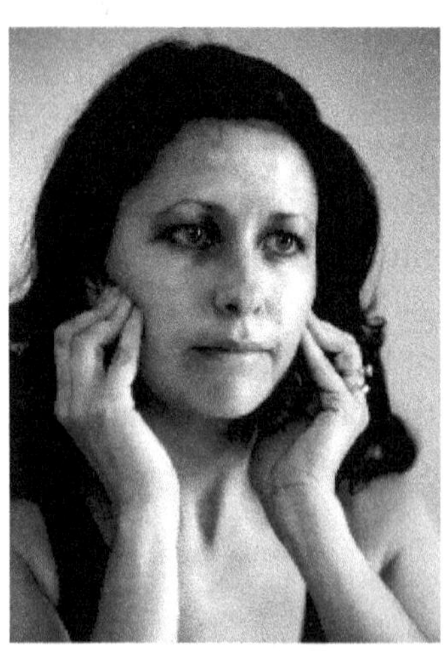

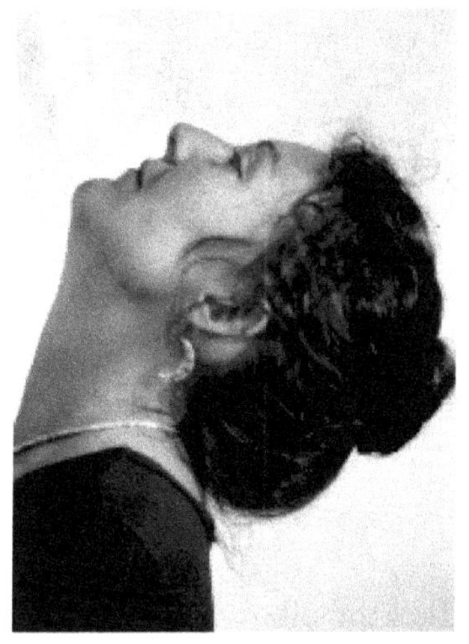

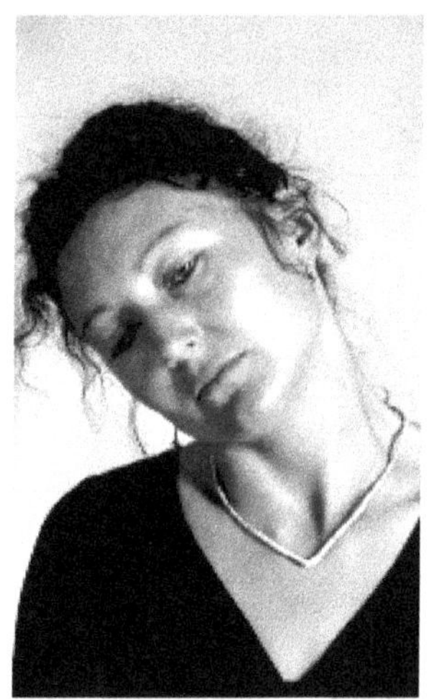

Neck: Move the neck back and forth, front, back and sideways. Turn the head to the left and right and completely around, circling left to right and right to left.

Shoulders: Using the arms, turn the shoulders from front to back and back to front. Then shake the arms up and down. Or you may lie face down on the floor, leaning on the arms, going up and down.

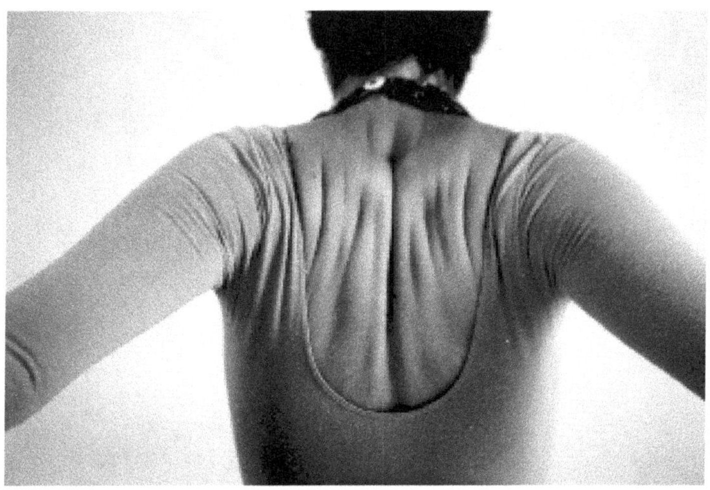

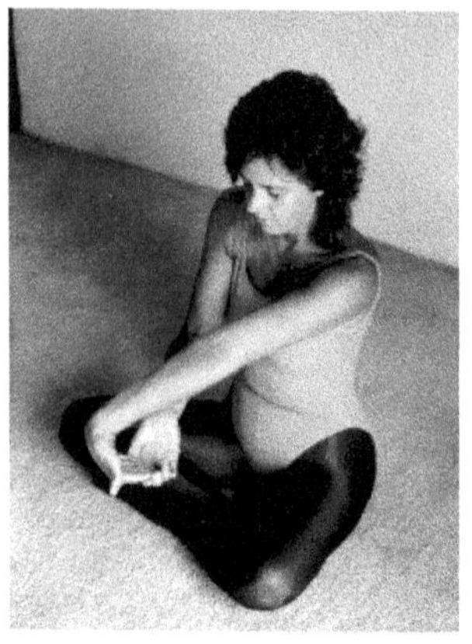

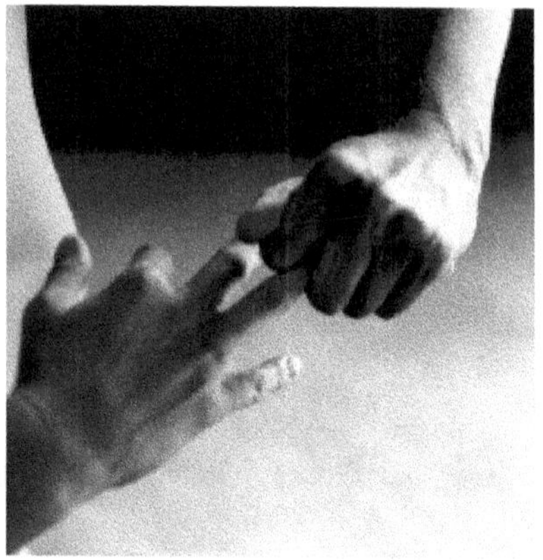

Arms and hands: Extend and flex the elbows, wrists and fingers. Twist and pull out the fingers. Twist the wrists, going up and down, sideways and around.

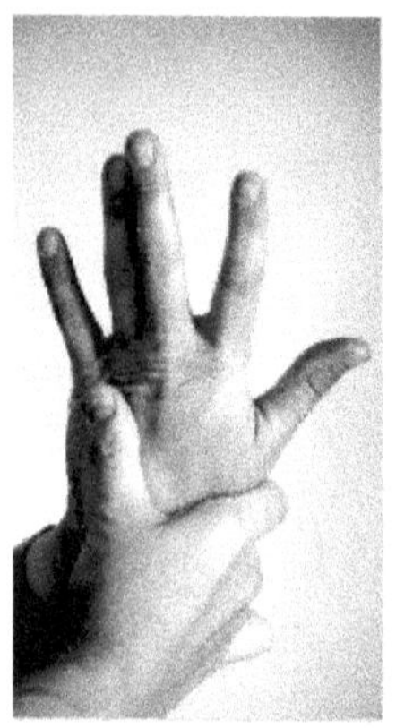

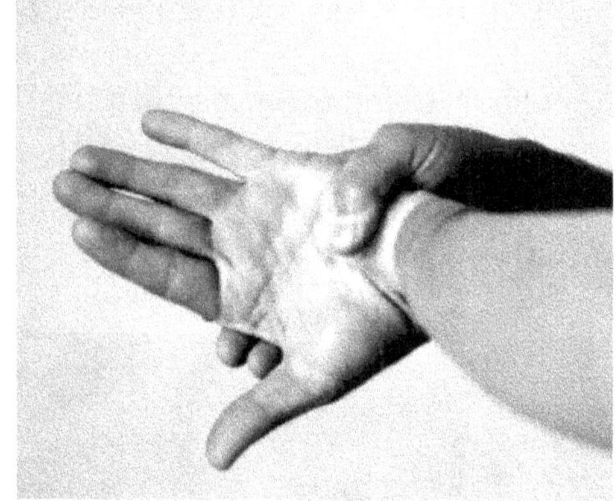

Chest: Push out the chest while inhaling and collapse at the end of expansion with a short exhale.

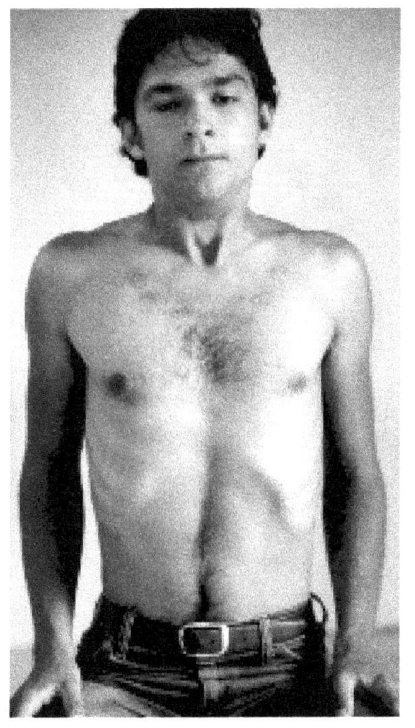

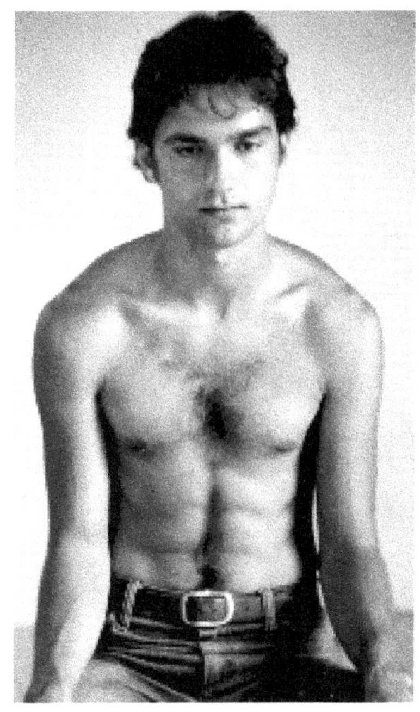

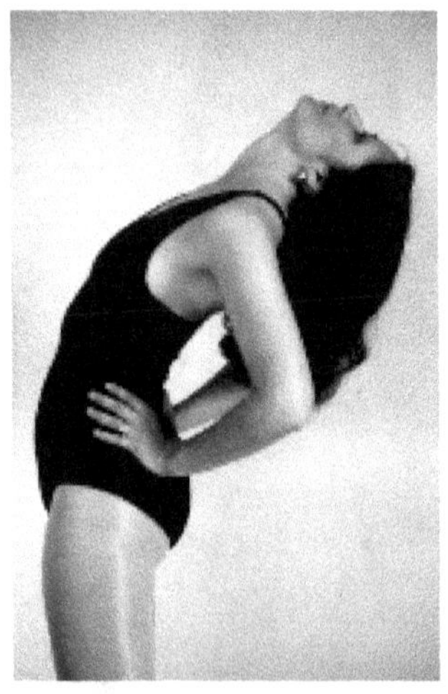

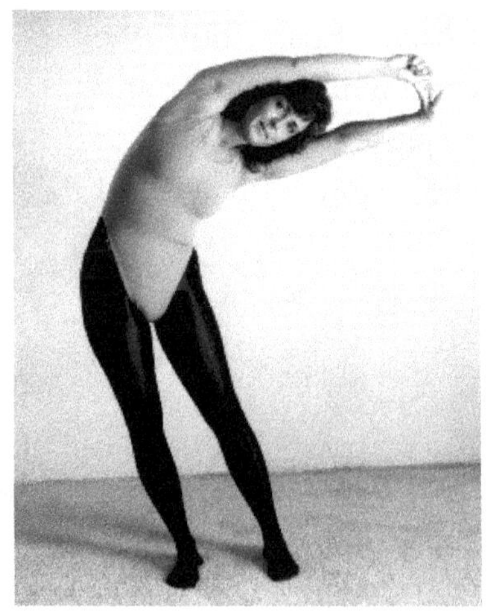

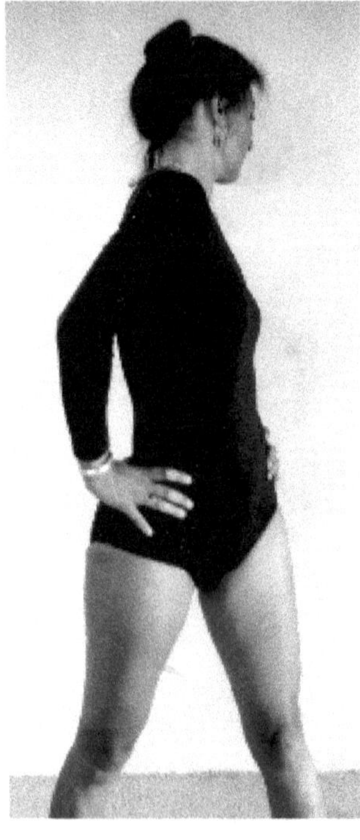

Sides of body: With hands on hips, bend up and down and sideways. Then twist the upper body from the waist, back and forth, and turn in a circular fashion, back and forth. This may also be done with the arms extended over the head.

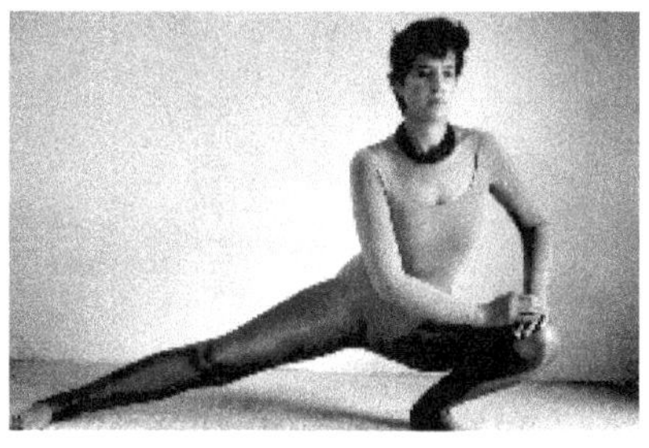

Thigh muscles and knees: Standing up, spread the legs and move from side to side, pulling the thigh muscles. With legs closer together, bend from the waist, back and front, twist back and forth, and turn in a circular fashion. Then stand up on the toes and bend the knees completely, going up and down.

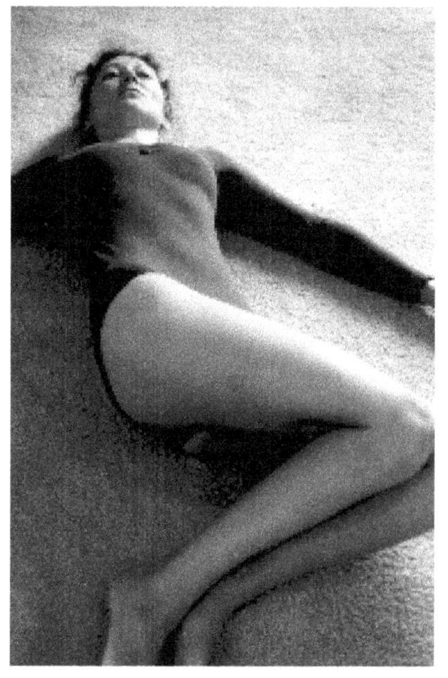

Abdomen, spine and hips: Breathing deeply from the abdomen, pull the abdomen up and down. Then move the belly around in a circle and in and out. Lie on your back, legs straight; sit up (inhaling) and come down (exhaling). Put the knees up and twist them from side to side. With legs straight, lie on your back and move back and forth like a goldfish.

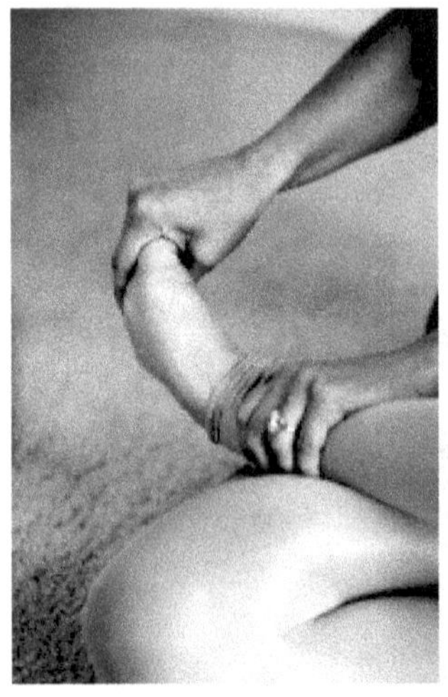
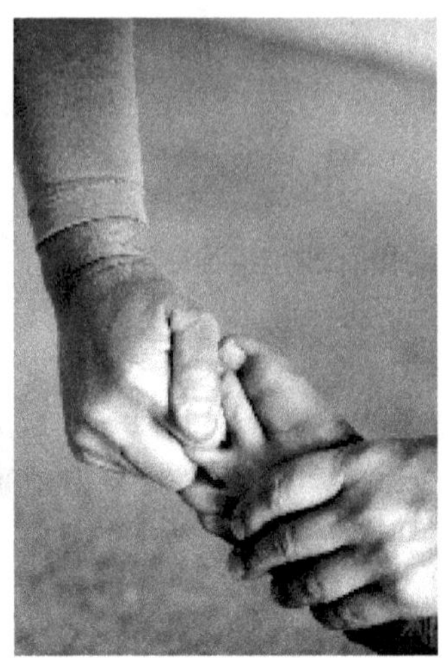

Ankles and toes: Crossing one leg over the other, twist the ankle, holding the ball of the foot. Turn the toes all together, then turn and pull one at a time.

These exercises may be done in the most comfortable position: sitting, standing, lying on the stomach, back or side. Be completely relaxed – no stiffness – and do not use any strength.

Any other exercises may be done according to the body's condition. You may do any kind of sport or daily work at home or business but do not force yourself or get too tired.

In our scientific civilization, much of the power of the body and spirit has been lost. It is absolutely necessary to slowly bring it back. Try to exercise all parts of the body as much as possible.

Very weak patients must be guided correctly and constantly diagnosed. Everything must be done gradually, slowly gaining strength. If forced too quickly, this condition might become dangerous; be very careful.

DIET AND PHYSICAL LIFE

Diet is the most important way to control physical life and activity. The wrong diet puts the entire body out of balance: cells, organs, etc. Sooner or later, the unbalanced circulation of energy causes illness. Those who are interested in studying natural therapy are obliged, first of all, to clearly understand this matter of diet.

The ability to have both physical and mental (or spiritual) activity manifests from the concentrating and expanding energies of the great center of the universe. The concentrating action of **WI** attracts all the formed and unformed energies necessary to the space of the body. By its force of gravity, it draws these energies and organizes them in the body. It converts them into other energies, such as when a grain of rice becomes a part of our blood cells.

Underlying this, the perfect creation of the body, is the action of the life will's judgment, **I-E**. It creates the body's constitution and the gravitational power of **WI** maintains it. **I-WI** is the human substance, front and back. The energy attracted by **WI** 's concentrating power is what is meant by diet. Diet is used here in its broadest sense; including heat, cold, air, etc. The life will converts all of these energies into spiritual and physical activity. Finally, it expands from the body's space and disappears.

All these energies that concentrate and expand from the human physical space have one source for the action of the human substance, **I-WI**. If the rhythms of these energies were separated, they would divide into **A-O-U-E-I**, the five dimensions of the mother sound rhythms:

1) The action of **A** dimension is the energy rhythm of human spiritual capacity.
2) **O** dimension manifests the rhythm of memory and knowledge.
3) **U** dimension is the material of the physical constitution which manifests the rhythms of the five physical senses.
4) **E** dimension is the action which manifests the rhythm of the capacity for judgment.

A-O-U-E are a priori dimensions; when manifest, they are four mother sounds. A priori manifests the capacity of a posteriori this way. Each one is a different dimension or rhythm of the action of life energy. Theoretical physics' energy dimensions (the grand unification or String Theory) really refers to these dimensions. They manifest directly through the human mouth as these vowel sounds. They converge and manifest a posteriori human capacity. The source of these dimensions is **I-WI**. The **I-WI** dimension is total universal creation which transforms itself into the action of the total finite and infinite universe.

The content of the universe's activity converts into human capacity and is its source point; it is the seed of the universe. Life will is **I** and life power is **WI**. This is how **A-O-U-E-I**, the five a priori dimensions of energy, act within a limited space, concentrating and expanding. In this space is created all human physical and spiritual capacity – complete human life. To keep this life in perfect condition – to allow it to realize its full potential – we must know the order of our life. We must maintain perfect balance of the body's five dimensions of energy. We begin by studying and searching the therapy principles evolved by our ancestors and follow their way.

It is too simple to speak only of the balance and synchronization of the dimensions. Each dimension has a front and back, expanding and concentrating. There are also the ways the dimensions' currents synchronize and relate to each other. Furthermore, each dimension behaves in terms of its eight motive vibrations (**T-K-M-H-L-N-Y-S**, the eight father rhythms). To keep all of these factors in harmony by trying to use scientific knowledge (**O** dimension) – by calculation, theory and measurement – is quite impossible. Yet without this harmony, the body becomes sick or its spiritual capacity is impaired. A sick condition inevitably creates our unhappiness and lack of freedom – a lifetime of suffering.

All human beings should know the basic method for achieving harmony. Some may feel it is a very difficult matter because it is not something which lends itself to scientific measurement. It is really very simple and so fundamental; scientific knowledge is unnecessary. It just means to return to the mother's embrace; going back to the breast of the natural universe. All we need to do is to follow the judgment of our inner substance, the life will within us.

The cause of the sickness of modern times is an erroneous source of knowledge. We must throw out everything we know. This is the first step toward building a pure, human civilization. First we must eat only natural food and know how to balance concentrating and expanding energies and the circulation of the five dimensions. We also need to do enough exercise from the time we are young, each of us developing to the maximum, physically and spiritually. We also need to live in a natural environment with clean air, earth and water.

HOW TO EAT

1. We must have natural food which grows in the local climate, and clean water. Grains are an exception and do not have to grow where you live.

2. Food should be chewed well, the more the better. Especially in the case of sick people, food must be completely masticated, reducing it to a pulp which is automatically swallowed.

3. The human substance **I-WI**, indicates through the number of teeth that we have, how to naturally harmonize with the order of the universe. It shows us the types and percentages of food necessary to us. In adults, there are twenty molars for grinding grains, eight incisors for cutting vegetables, and four canines for chewing meat.

Percentages of types of food:

a) Adult (32 teeth)
Grains 20/32 = 62.5%
Vegetables 8/32 = 25%
Animal protein 4/32 = 12.5%

b) Pre-adult (28 teeth)
Grains 16/28 = 57%
Vegetables 8/28 = 29%
Animal protein 4/28 = 14%

c) Older child (24 teeth)
Grains 12/24 = 50%
Vegetables 8/24 = 33%
Animal protein 4/24 = 17%

d) Young child (20 teeth)
Grains 8/20 = 40%
Vegetables 8/20 = 40%
Animal protein 4/20 = 20%

Food and drink are one part of the concentrating energy we receive from outside for maintaining balance. The food we eat has its own life energy which is concentrating and expanding. The contents of the food's inner energy, according to type and within the same type, have different powers of concentration and expansion: larger, smaller, stronger, weaker, longer, shorter, etc. To have a long and healthy life, we must take in those foods which have elements and cells of long duration, that is, which have more concentrating energy.

The choice of food is made, finally, from the judgment of **I-WI**. Before this, however, each person is influenced by family tradition, habits and personal tastes; or from his/her knowledge and understanding. The quantity and choice of what one eats will vary with the individual.

I-WI's judgment can take the necessary elements only from what is presented to it; the actual food being ingested. The life will's judgment manifests through the physical senses of **U** and the experience of **O**. The desires of **U-O** dimension do not directly manifest **I-WI**. Habits, tastes, local conditions and knowledge (such as aspirin for colds and vitamins for energy) influence what action is taken. The desires and judgment of **U-O** separate from the life will **I-WI**, which leads to a great error in the kinds of food and drink which are preferred.

As I said, **I-WI** creates all the elements and cells necessary to the body's system and arranges them in perfect order, in the space of the body. It keeps it in perfect condition, giving the body its life action. **U-O** should follow what is being asked by the substance and choose only the right kinds of food and drink. But **U-O** does not obey the inner voice. It acts independently, making its own choice, which sooner or later causes the body to lose its balance and strength. This matter becomes clearer when you compare the difference in life capacity between wild animals and their domesticated breeds.

The concentrating power of some food and drinks is strong – their elements have greater strength and longer life span – and some have just the opposite nature.

COMPARISON OF FRUITS AND GRAINS

1. The most concentrating power in fruit is found in the seeds and skin. Balancing with this strong concentration is the rest of the fruit, in which the elements are almost totally expansive. This is the part we eat, so in order to create new body cells, **I-WI** is obliged to choose elements from the expanding side of the fruit alone.

2. Grains also have a balance of elements, but the action of expansion has not yet begun; all their energy is being held in concentration. When we eat grains, it is from these concentrating elements that **I-WI** sorts out what it needs to create new cells.

The body is constantly creating new cells from the food it ingests, but the strength of its life power varies according to the kind of food it uses. For instance, red blood cells clearly have different levels of strength depending on what is ingested, even though they are all the same type of cell. There is no question which person's cell structure has stronger and more enduring life power; that person has a stronger, healthier and longer life.

Each formed life must have a balance of both concentrating and expanding energies, but the power of its gravity center will last over different lengths of time. When the seed is being formed, concentration is stronger, but only in the space of the seed. The expanding energy separates to the outer area around the seed, and elements collected from there to make new body cells are obliged to have a shorter and weaker life span. The bones and tendons of a child's body are soft (expansive) so that the concentrating energy must separate from expansion to strengthen them. The body, during childhood, has concentrating and expanding energies which are equally strong. As it matures, the bones harden and are less flexible, and expanding energy goes to its other parts. In old age, the body is less concentrating and expands more, losing strength and developing wrinkles, flabbiness, etc.

FOOD CATEGORIES

1. **Grains**: The plant's total life potential is here in one seed. If conditions are not present for sprouting, it can survive for thousands of years, still maintaining life. The concentrating energy received from this type of food is therefore the strongest and most enduring for the human body.

2. **Vegetables**: We eat either the leaves, stems or roots of vegetables; we almost never have its whole life. Expanding elements are mostly in the leaves and stalks, which are balanced with the concentrating elements in the roots. We, however, usually consume only one side of a plant's energy.

3. **Animal protein** (meat and animal products): The elements and cells from this dimension of physical life are transmuted from those of the plant world. Most of the concentrating elements' energy is in the bones, tendons, skin and hair. To balance with this, expanding energy is mostly in the blood, fat and muscles. The flesh, where the expanding energy is located, is what we usually eat.

The contents of each animal's milk are designed to serve that kind of animal's capacity; the cells contain the elements needed for each animal's type of body. All kinds of milk are considered to be high in nutrition; it can be judged scientifically which milk is superior and which inferior. What science cannot see is the life world, and from their research, they jump to the conclusion that since animal's milk is so rich, it is also a superior drink for the human body.

In reality, the qualities of cow milk make it the most desirable drink for a calf; that of goats for kids and sheep for lambs. Cow milk can never be better for a kid than the mother goat's milk. For the adult cow, natural grasses are a better food than cow milk. If a cow is sick, it would be nonsense to try to make it well by giving it cow milk, or goat or sheep milk. From the viewpoint of natural therapy, it would be an insane thing to do. Yet it is this insanity which passes for human knowledge in our society. It is a widely accepted theory of nutrition, held strongly in the minds of most people all over the world; this is most people's **O** dimension understanding.

It is the convention for the human mother to stop nursing early and supplant her milk with cow's or goat's milk for her children. As I explained, it is the life will and energy of the cow that creates its milk; the contents of goat's milk are the result of a goat's life energy; a dog's milk is a dog's energy, etc. At the bottom of each animal's milk is the life will and energy of its a posteriori life. The action of its a priori life will and energy cannot be separated from the contents of each animal's milk, different for each one. The life will and energy of a cow continues to act inside its milk.

A human mother hands over her own life will and energy, with all her warmth and tenderness. She also hands over her emotional sense along with the life energy of her milk and this is transmitted to the baby. Why should she forsake this great responsibility in order to follow an insane convention?

I am not just talking about milk, although I used it as an example of animal food. At the bottom of the contents of such food is that animal's life will. Whatever animal we eat: birds, fish, eggs, beef, etc., its constitution becomes the contents of the elements and cells of our body. Each animal's life will and energy are there.

4. **Fruit**: As previously explained, we eat that part of the fruit which has strongly expanding energy elements. If we eat fruit frequently, it weakens our cells, shortening their life. Fruit, because of its strongly expanding and separating energy, is needed for a heavy meat eater, in order to clean out the poisons found in meat. It is not possible, however, to measure the precise amount necessary to do just this and not so much that the cells are destroyed.

People native to a tropical country eat some amount of fruit in order to balance the heat of the sun, but they cannot eat so much. They are already in harmony with the environment in which they were born and raised. If people native to a cold climate were to move to the tropics, they would need to eat a much greater quantity of fruit there.

5. **Drinks**:

a) Alcohol has a strongly expanding energy which helps purify the body of poisons. It is especially needed for those on a predominantly meat diet; a certain quantity may be regarded as medicinal. Alcohol is not needed at all for those on a diet of vegetables and grains. Given the conditions of a tropical country such as southern India where the population is strictly vegetarian, alcohol is poison.

b) Water must be clean and natural, without too great a mineral content. Too much water is not desirable.

6. **Condiments**: The quantity and types used should be in harmony with the climate and geographical location of where one lives, as well as the season it is. For instance, in a hot climate or high altitude, hot foods such as chili are necessary.

a) Salt is the most important condiment and should be made from natural sea water. Salt that has been processed to make it white is not desirable.

b) Sugar: Traditionally it is said that sugar is totally poisonous and of absolutely no benefit. It is better not to use it at all. If some sweets are really necessary and it is either a tropical or temperate climate, one can use a little natural black sugar or honey. In wintertime or in an arctic climate, sweets are not needed at all. White, refined sugar is absolutely forbidden.

From ancient times, the traditional preparation of condiments has had a deep and important meaning. They can be useful but too much can be dangerous. We must know how to use them according to each person's condition.

7. **Commercial Food**: Any prepared food and drinks which have artificial additives (often used to enhance color and smell) are absolutely forbidden to use. Those which have been naturally processed, such as by drying, can be used in a limited quantity. They cannot be a main source of food because processing has diminished their life energy.

From the recommended types of food and drinks I have already outlined, one should choose what one needs in order to perfectly harmonize with the conditions of here and now. Type and quantity should be judged exactly as to that place, the day and time. For the human being, the time of eating and drinking is a most serious moment. It is the moment which decides what our future life and fortune will be; how our capacity shall be fulfilled. It should be as a ceremony, with respect for the life will and with thanks for this way of receiving our a posteriori capacity.

The right kind and quantity of food and drink is finally decided by our highest judgment, the human life will **I-WI**. This decision cannot be made by using **O** dimension knowledge and the **U** dimension desires of the five physical senses; it is impossible to know what choice to make when judging from there. The highest judgment measures the body's inner energy, expanding and concentrating, taking into account our a posteriori physical and spiritual activities, and knows how much of each energy requires replenishment. This is measured in relation to outside energies (light, heat, air, etc.) or to the conditions of synchronization prior to this. The synchronizing and exchanging that occur between human physical life energy and total universal energy, changing from second to second, evolving and disappearing – all those conditions are caught exactly, are taken into account and judged. To keep the body in perfect harmony with the rest of the universe, the amount and type of food and drink is chosen for that day, that time and place. It is impossible to know this by scientific calculation. That way is too far removed from the decision of this dimension's world.

This highest judgment is the decision of the human life will which gives the a posteriori five physical senses that which it senses and desires. We feel thirsty, hungry, tired, sleepy, etc., and we want to do something about it. This is how the life will manifests in a posteriori and it is most important to be careful of how those desires are met. We should not mistakenly satisfy them from **O** dimension scientific knowledge or personal, past experience. The mistakes of the past become habits, and we should not satisfy the desires of bad habits.

When thirsty, just drink clean, natural water and the life will shall say, "Yes! Good! Enough!" At the same time, the tongue, mouth and stomach, and all the desires of the physical senses will feel satisfied; that is the way it is with the natural, human body. When we are guided by **U-O** dimensions' desires, we prefer to have coca-cola or beer. When we are hungry, we remember some tasty food we had before and want some more.

We do not realize how much our mistakes disturb the body later on; we do not know how to reflect about it. When we have taken the wrong kind and quantity of food and drink, that part of the body or the body's total condition must be affected to some degree; there will be some loss of balance. When we have taken the wrong energy, the life will tells us about it through the five physical senses and the five spiritual senses. If, however, the experience is not too painful, it is quickly forgotten. We continue making the same mistake and, more and more, we wish only to have a nice taste in the mouth, refusing to listen to the inner voice of our life will. Sometimes, we feel something is not good to have, but we are so attracted by the taste that we can easily ignore that right feeling. This means we no longer have the fear of God.

From whatever we eat and drink, the body receives some quantity of energy which should then be expanded for it to stay in harmony. When the body is filled with energy, the judgment of the life will is to spend it. It orders us to do some type of spiritual or physical action; that is how the desire for action is made manifest. As I have said, the action taken can be the wrong one, out of ignorance or folly or mistaken information from the experienced desires of **U-O** dimension. We do not follow our substance's command, **I-E** dimension. This kind of blind **U-O** dimension action causes what effect on the body? Clearly it is shown to us if we can but understand it.

Most people's decisions are based on scientific knowledge, **U-O** dimension; this is the way of actual civilization. People do not pay attention to the orders of their life will **I-WI**, which created their physical life. Not only are our lives sacrificed this way, but decisions and understandings based on **U-O** create all the misery there is on earth; call it the way of Satan. The substance of Satan is our own lower dimensions' judgment and the acts which stem from those desires. We should clearly be aware of this. I shout this truth in my loudest voice and though I can be heard, my voice has not yet penetrated people's hearts.

I have already said this in so many ways: the cause of spiritual and physical sickness is ignorance of the a priori universe's creation, the life will **I** and the life force **WI**, which manifests the a posteriori human beings' total capacity. One cannot recognize this truth by one's self or have any knowledge of it, so that, unconsciously, the absolute law of life is disobeyed and there is no escaping retribution. It is worse than a robot turning against its creator. For our mental and physical actions to be in perfect harmony, we must simply follow the orders of our inner substance, **I-WI**. To explain **I-WI** in depth, however, is not so simple. This is an explanation of just one part of it, the part most immediate to our daily lives, that is, diet – the right way of food and drink.

Diet, of course, is not all that creates the proper conditions for perfect health and the ability to fully realize one's self. Yet, to be healthy and to treat an illness, diet is a most important consideration. In your daily life, you must go more deeply and come completely face to face with your substance. Then your life shall be guided perfectly by the highest dimension of your life will, **I-WI**.

I have become completely confident about this. Today, I just try to live a natural life, leaving everything to the direct judgment and desire of my substance. If my body becomes sick, it means I could not listen to the absolute order of my substance. My reflection was not deep enough nor my self-purification adequate. Perhaps I had heard it well enough but I was pulled down by my lower dimensions' desires, i.e., the devil spirit; I had not been mindful of my absolute orders. In any case, it was my own crime against myself. I must totally accept whatever mental or physical distress I am in as the punishment of my life will. I continue to live this way, with gratitude and apologies to my substance.

8. **Some Diet Drinks**

a) Three-year Bancha tea (from a natural food store).

b) Brown rice tea: wash rice and dry roast until dark brown. Store it, and, when needed, boil some and drink.

c) Wheat and varieties of wheat tea: same as rice tea.

d) Diet coffee: dry roast red azuki beans and soy beans to a dark brown, resembling coffee beans. Grind to a flour and add hot (boiled) water to drink.

e) Kombu tea: wash and dry the kombu, then grind to a powder. Store it. Add hot (boiled) water to drink.

9. **Therapeutic Drinks**

a) Ume Sho Bancha: to prepare, make three-year bancha tea. Add one large umeboshi (pitted) or two small ones and one third that amount grated ginger. Add one tablespoon soy sauce to eight ounces of bancha. Mix and drink.

b) Kuzu, porridge or soup: dissolve kuzu in a little cold water, adding a little grated ginger and soy sauce. Stirring quickly, add boiling water until mixture becomes transparent. How thick or thin this should be depends on the person's condition.

Both a) and b) may be used for all conditions.

c) Radish water: wash a daikon, leaving on the skin. Grate three tablespoons of daikon; add ten percent of that amount grated ginger and one and a half tablespoons soy sauce; mix. Add one and a half cups very hot bancha tea. Drink all at once.

This is powerfully effective for an inner fever from a cold or for a chilled feeling; it aids in perspiration. After drinking this, go to bed and cover up until you have completely sweated it out. Wash up and change to dry clothes and bedding. This is absolutely forbidden for a weak person, particularly with a heart condition. Even a very strong person cannot do this more than twice.

d) Chamomile tea: this is for a weak person needing more concentrating energy.

e) Osha: this is only for a strong person needing expanding energy.

f) Apple juice: this is an expanding energy drink, not to be used for a person with weak concentrating energy.

g) Other herbal teas: you must know the nature of each herb or you can make the condition worse.

SOME SIMPLE REMEDIES

a) Hot ginger compress: grate about 112.5 grams (four ounces) of ginger root, older ones are preferable, into a cloth bag and tie it up. Dip the bag into a half liter (about one quart) of boiling water and squeeze, making the water a pale yellow; darker is not necessary. Keep the water warm on a low fire. Place a towel into the water and gently squeeze it out, in order to avoid burning the skin. Apply the towel to the abnormal area so as to warm it up (placing another cover on top). You may also rub the towel back and forth over the area.

This is an expanding energy which helps make the blood circulate more smoothly, eliminating blood clots. It therefore helps stiffness or painfulness of the shoulder (contraction), cyst of the breast (contraction), nervous condition, skin sores, bruises.

b) Arbi paste (taro root): remove skin and grate. Add the same amount of whole wheat flour, ten percent grated ginger root and enough water to mix into a paste. Make the paste three quarters of a centimeter (1/4 to 3/8 of an inch) thick and place into a paper or cloth. Apply the paste after a ginger compress application (see above) and change the paste every five or six hours, warming the area with a ginger compress between paste applications.

If prolonged use is necessary, the skin may become irritated. After a ginger application, dry the skin and rub in sesame oil. Do not allow the skin to become overly irritated.

This paste affects the activity of concentrating and expanding energy, a little more on the expanding side. It can help such problems as cancer, swellings (cysts, etc.), rheumatism, burnt skin and all pain from skin inflammation. Arbi root is also available as a prepared powder which is more convenient to store. Simply add water to make the paste and apply as above.

c) Vegetable paste: this can be substituted for arbi. Grind green vegetable leaves and mix with ten percent grated ginger and enough wheat flour to make into the consistency of bread dough. This affects pain from inflammation and takes away fever; as an exterior application.

d) Tofu paste: squeeze the water from tofu through a cloth. Mix in about twenty percent wheat flour to make a paste about three quarters of a centimeter thick (1/4 to 3/8 in.). Put into a cloth and apply; change every two hours. Takes away fever from the head, chest and abdomen.

e) Mustard paste: make a paste from ground mustard seeds. If using mustard powder, add thirty percent wheat flour and enough water to make a paste. Apply. It takes away fever.

f) Meat paste: use one to two centimeters thick red meat. Apply. It is also used to take away fever.

g) Apple juice: juice fresh apples and apply; for fever from a headache.

h) Daikon juice: grate a daikon and squeeze out the juice. Apply. For headache, chapped and bleeding skin and inflammation from a bruise.

i) Lotus root juice: grate a fresh lotus root, squeezing out the juice. To two tablespoons lotus root juice add one teaspoon ginger root juice and a little natural salt. Add four ounces of hot water and drink three times daily. For a cough and catarrh of the throat.

j) Raw brown rice: every morning, while you are still hungry (before eating or drinking anything), chew a handful of raw rice very well, until it is a pulp. Used to clean out worms.

k) Salt bancha: add one percent salt to bancha tea. Use to wash the eyes and nose.

l) For burns, immediately cool the area with salt water until the pain stops. Apply sesame oil. You may also apply arrowroot juice.

m) Ume Extract: this may be purchased at a natural food store. Always use in small doses. To strengthen the stomach and intestines; it corresponds to the digestive organs. It is powerful in protecting the body from contagious diseases such as cholera and typhoid fever. In an epidemic, take beforehand as a preventative measure.

If already contracted and there is a fever, take ume and it will be cured within two or three days. In summer, if the water is bad, mix in a little ume to protect against viruses.

n) Miso oil: to prepare, boil up about four ounces of black sesame oil, adding 375 grams of natural miso, cooking slowly over a low fire. Stir constantly until miso is completely dissolved in the oil; it should darken. Keep it on the table and use a little with every meal. White sesame oil is a substitute but not as effective. It helps with a weak concentrating condition: heart disease, rheumatism, arthritis, near and far sightedness, tired eyes and all eye problems.

o) Egg Yolk: use only fertilized eggs. Separate the raw yolk from the white, as well as the cell. Add two or three drops of natural soy sauce and swallow in one gulp! It is used for weak, concentrating/overactive expanding condition of heart disease. Use only in an emergency when the heart is pumping too much and it is difficult to breathe. Can only be used twice a day. Do not use commercial, unfertilized eggs because they do not help and their poisons may make the condition worse.

COMPARATIVE CHART OF YIN/YANG

Devising this Yin/Yang chart was very difficult because in order to make it perfect, one must search the basic life rhythms inside one's own body – at the bottom of physical life. They must then be compared with the Kototama Fifty Sound Principle. To write scientifically about the a priori and a posteriori matters thus grasped has been a difficult task indeed.

This chart shows how the life action of concentration and expansion of the universe manifest phenomena in terms of daily food and drink. Studying and practicing with this chart as a comparison will help you to open your highest dimension's inner judgment, **I-E**. That means, opening your Eye of Life.

SUBJECT	YIN NATURE		YANG NATURE
Kototama Sound	WA		A
Life Action	attraction		expansion
	gravity		separation
	concentration		
Mother Sounds	U, O	I	E, A
Gogio - 5 Elements	earth, water	fire	metal, wood
Space	earth	human	heaven
Direction	north		south
	west		east
	coming down		going up
	right to left		left to right
Season	autumn		spring
	winter		summer
Time	night		day
	evening		morning
Dimension	time		space
Poisons	cold, dry	wet	heat, wind
Environment	land		sea
	lower land		higher land
	inland		beach
Light Rays	ultra-violet		infra-red
Element	carbon		oxygen
	sodium		potassium
	calcium		magnesium
pH	alkaline		acid
Vitamin	A, D, E, F, K		C, B, B-12, P
Compactness	small		large
Weight	heavy, dense		light
Form	small		large
	short		long
Emotion	sad	peaceful	angry

SUBJECT	YIN NATURE		YANG NATURE
Emotion	melancholy	peaceful	happy
Mental Activity	spiritual		materialistic
	religion		politics
	philosophy		economics
	art		business
	loner		sociable
	introvert		extrovert
Presence	outside yin		outside yang
	inside yang		inside yin
	slow		fast
	hard		soft
Physical Activity	immobile		mobile
	inactive		active
	slow		speedy
Social Action	peace		war
Life Forms	woman		man
	feminine		masculine
	plant		animal
Mental Action	quiet, inactive		loud, active
	negative		positive
Longevity	long life		short life
Respiration	inhalation		exhalation
Age	old, middle	young	childhood
	age	adult	infancy
Physical Strength	endurance		short span
Form	solid		liquid
	liquid		air
	oil		air
	oil		water
More Active In	fall		spring
	winter		summer
	night-time		daytime

SUBJECT	YIN NATURE	YANG NATURE
Temperature	cold	hot
	cool	warm
Food	grain	vegetable
	grain	animal protein
	vegetable	animal protein
	animal protein	fruit
	seed	grain
	grain	nuts
	root vegetables	leafy vegetables
	dried food	raw food
	cooked food	raw food
Plants	tubers, grasses	tall plants
Taste	acrid, puckering	sweet, sour, hot
	bitter	acid
	salty	acid
Color	black	white
	violet	yellow
	indigo	orange
	blue	red
	green	crimson
Animal World	egg, shellfish fish	animal, bird
Condiments	salt	sugar
	salt	vinegar
	sugar	vinegar
Drinks	natural water	juices
	natural water	vinegar
	vinegar	alcoholic drinks
	natural water	soda, juice
	natural water	alcohol
	soda, juice	alcohol

SUBJECT	YIN NATURE	YANG NATURE
Cooking Time	slow cooking	fast cooking
	boiling slowly	boiling quickly
Facial Form	△ □ ○	▯ ▽
Eyes	small	large
	pupil below	pupil above
	upper white	lower white
	shows	shows
	upper sanpaku	lower sanpaku
	yonpaku (4 corner	
	white) pupil in center,	
	surrounded by white	
Ears	small	large
	thick	thin
	flat	protruding
	lower position	upper position
	long lobe	no lobe
Nose	thin, straight, pinched	flat, large, pug
Mouth and Lips	small	big
	thin	full
	tight	protruding
Body	muscular, short, big	tall, small muscles,
	bones, stocky	fat, tissues
Hair	black	red
	bushy, thick	thin
	brunette	light reddish, blond
	maintaining hair	losing hair

ABOUT THE AUTHOR

Hinomoto no Mikoto Masahilo Nakazono

O Sensei Nakazono devoted his entire life's energy pursuing the way to the final truth. This quest took him to near perfection of the traditional martial arts; years of rigorous spiritual practices; and decades of testing, questioning and perfecting all aspects of traditional oriental therapies. It led him to Ueshiba Sensei and mastery of Aikido; to Professor Ohsawa and the practice of Macrobiotics; to Sakai Sensei, the master of healing with the hands; and to Ogasawara Sensei, who guided him toward understanding the Kototama Principle.

This lifetime pursuit to grasp a unified understanding of the universe has resulted in a practical basis of health care.

Born in Kagoshima District, southern Japan, in 1918, Sensei Nakazono's earliest experiences of healing came from his mother, a nurse-midwife who used foods, herbs, poultices and massage in her work. She was highly respected and widely recognized for her ability to turn breech babies and demand for her services continued throughout his childhood.

His study of Kendo began at age six. Before his teens, Sensei began concentrating on the practice of Judo and began intensive professional studies when he was 14. By 1933, he earned his Black Belt in Judo and a year later began a two-year apprenticeship in the study and practice of Acupuncture with Dr. Juzo Motoyama in Nagasaki. In 1938, he received his license as a "Bone-Setter," an osteopathic specialty in structural repair and manipulation available only to instructors who had undergone specific rigorous training.

He was trained in Aikido, a martial art for self-purification, by its founder, Ueshiba Sensei. During the 1960s, he was the World Aikido Federation representative to Europe and North Africa and Director of the European Aikido Federation.

It was Ueshiba Sensei who introduced him to the Kototama Principle, saying it was the foundation of the principles of Aikido. However, Ueshiba Sensei continued to use the traditional metaphors and symbols by way of explanation and his teaching of the Unified World appeared theoretical or metaphysical. There were to be 18 more years of searching before Sensei Nakazono would come in contact with Ogasawara Sensei.

A professor named George Ohsawa developed some interesting nutritional ideas which he termed "Macrobiotics." Sensei Nakazono's association with Professor Ohsawa began in 1950 and their close relationship lasted over ten years. In 1955, Sensei left Japan and traveled to India where he established the Universal Institute. There he treated mental and physical disorders using Ohsawa's system; i.e., he diagnosed according to Macrobiotic theory and personally prepared each of his patient's meals. He treated there in this manner for three years. Upon his return to Japan, he was introduced to the renowned master of handwork therapy, Sakai Sensei. Master Sakai taught Sensei his own method: Te A Te (Spiritual Hand Treatment) and continued to guide him until his death. It was Master Sakai who fully grasped the spirit of finite form – Jizo Bosatsu. This "treatment by spirit" led Sakai Sensei to unique diagnostic powers and treatment methods which he passed on to Sensei Nakazono.

The first Aikido dojo outside of Japan was founded by Sensei in 1958, in Singapore. In 1960, he was a martial arts consultant to the government of South Vietnam.

In France, where he settled with his family in the early 1960s, he established the Kan Nagara Institute and began training European students in Aikido and therapy techniques. He traveled throughout Europe and North Africa during his 11 years in France. When he departed for the United States in 1972, he had over 40,000 European Aikido students and student practitioners of Natural Therapy.

The study of the Kototama Principle began when he established contact with Ogasawara Sensei. Though his teacher was in Japan and he was in France, the effect of his studies and the correspondences between teacher and student transformed his life – thoughts, speech, Aikido, therapy work – all dimensions underwent profound transformation. Kototama meditation became Kototama life. The movements of Aikido changed, viewpoints changed, the understanding of Natural Therapy changed and its application took on an entirely new meaning.

A six-month visit to the U.S. in 1970 resulted in his decision to establish a center of learning in Santa Fe, New Mexico. In 1972, he arrived in Santa Fe, opened a medical clinic and dojo and began teaching Aikido and Oriental Medicine as manifestations of the Kototama Principle.

Weekly discourses on the Kototama Principle began and publishing efforts were initiated; students increased and the load at his clinic grew. In January 1973, patients of Sensei introduced an Acupuncture Practice Act in the State Senate. This was the first acupuncture legislation ever considered in the United States.

His healing capacities became widely known and it was necessary for him to ask his son, Katsuharu K. Nakazono Sensei, to come to Santa Fe and assist him. His son, also a highly ranked Aikido master and Acupuncturist, arrived in Santa Fe in 1974. By 1977, he and his son had treated well over 4,000 patients who came from all parts of the country and various parts of the world seeking his unique methods of treatment. His patient waiting list grew, people were waiting two months to be seen and it was decided to teach Kototama Life Medicine on a formal basis. In the fall of 1978, he enrolled his first class at the Kototama Institute.

The Kototama Institute provided a formal education in the basics of traditional Acupuncture, a post-graduate clinical program in Kototama Life Medicine and a ten-year doctoral program for those seeking to be Doctors of Kototama Life Medicine.

Sensei Nakazono was a consultant to the Hawaiian Acupuncture Board, and was widely read in Japanese professional journals. In the spring of 1985, he returned to France at the invitation of the French Osteopathic Association and the French Aikido Federation as a guest lecturer.

In 1984, Santa Fe citizens bestowed on him the award, "Living Treasure of Santa Fe." During the 1985 Legislative session, the New Mexico State Senate honored Sensei Nakazono with the Award of Exceptional Achievement "for having inspired and directed the passage of the New Mexico Acupuncture Act, for having established schools and for the professional practice and recognition of acupuncture in this State since 1972."

Through his classes, his patients and his writings, Sensei Nakazono has asked the world to seriously study the Kototama Principle. It is for all humanity. This is the message of his life's work.

PRACTICING SOUNDS

Practice begins with the pronunciation of the sounds aloud. When meditating, breathe slowly, making each breath as long as possible. Breath deeply from the tanden (a point just below the navel) – not from the chest.

Make the sound of ***SU*** and then ***A-WA***. Do not use any technique or decoration, such as a melody. Just let the sounds come out naturally; otherwise, you are beginning with an intellectual action and you will not be able to see anymore.

To make sounds is an action of expansion. It should start from the point of final concentration, the absolute center. That is why all Kana sounds always start with the teeth held firmly together.

The rhythm of sounds, our life's manifestation, is based on ***I*** dimension, the life will. When making the ***I*** sounds, the teeth remain closed; they are always made by biting the teeth.

A-O-U-E, the four dimensions of mother sounds, and the child sounds, come out from ***I***. With each sound, always return to biting the teeth.

A sound is energy expanding to the fullest and made with a fully opened mouth. ***O*** sound is made with a round mouth, half closed; the smallest opening comes out as ***U*** sound. ***I*** and ***E*** sounds are made with the mouth open sideways. The teeth open for ***E*** but remain closed for ***I***.

It is the same inner energy that is expanding; only the form of the mouth changes. Our human life energy can expand in only these five ways – these five sounds.

When making the *WA* sounds, say ***U-U-U-WA***; you can see it better that way. Try to see the difference between the light of *A* and *WA*. There is no shrine or ceremony that uses only one candle. There are always two lights which symbolize the manifestation of human capacity and *A* and *WA*.

TAKAAMA HALA NI MOTOTUMI O YASUME OHO KAMI ▪ AMATANO KA MI GAMI WO TUDOYETE ▪ TOKO TO WA NI KA MI TU MA LI MASU ▪ KAMULOGI KAMULOMI NO MIKOTO MOTITE ▪ KAMU IZANAGI NO MIKOTO ▪ TUKUSI NO HI MUKA NO TATI HANANO ▪ ODO NO AHAGI GA HALA NI MISOGI HALAI TAMOU TO KINI ▪ NALI MASELU HALAIDO NO OHOKAMI TATI ▪ MOLO MOLO NO MAGAKOTO TU MI KEGALE WO ALAZI TO ▪ HALAI TAMAE KIYOME TAMAE TO MOUSU ▪

KOTONO YOSI WO ▪ AMATUKAMI KUNI TU KAMI ▪ YAO YO LOZU NO KAMITATI TOMONI ▪ AMENO FUTI KOMA NO MI MI FULI TATETE KIKO SIME SE TO ▪ KASI KOMI KASI KOMI MO MO SUU ▪

KAM NAGALA TAMATI HAIYE MASE ▪ KAM NAGALA TAMATI HAIYE MASE ▪ KAM NAGALA TAMATI HAIYE MASE ▪

金木
KANAGI

わ ら や ま は な た さ か あ
WA LA YA MA HA NA TA SA KA A

ゐ り い み ひ に ち し き い
WI LI YI MI HI NI TI SI KI I

う る ゆ む ふ ぬ つ す く う
WU LU YU MU HU NU TU SU KU U

ゑ れ え め へ ね て せ け え
WE LE YE ME HE NE TE SE KE E

を ろ よ も ほ の と そ こ お
WO LO YO MO HO NO TO SO KO O

WN

菅曽
SUGASO

ワ ナ ラ マ ヤ ハ サ カ タ ア
WA NA LA MA YA HA SA KA TA A

ヲ ノ ロ モ ヨ ホ ソ コ ト オ
WO NO LO MO YO HO SO KO TO O

ウ ヌ ル ム ユ フ ス ク ツ ウ
WU NU LU MU YU HU SU KU TU U

ヱ ネ レ メ エ ヘ セ ケ テ エ
WE NE LE ME YE HE SE KE TE E

ヰ ニ リ ミ イ ヒ シ キ チ イ
WI NI LI MI YI HI SI KI TI I

AN

太祝詞
FUTONOLITO

ワ サ ヤ ナ ラ ハ マ カ タ ア
WA SA YA NA LA HA MA KA TA A

ヰ シ イ ニ リ ヒ ミ キ チ イ
WI SI YI NI LI HI MI KI TI I

ヱ セ エ ネ レ ヘ メ ケ テ エ
WE SE YE NE LE HE ME KE TE E

ヲ ソ ヨ ノ ロ ホ モ コ ト オ
WO SO YO NO LO HO MO KO TO O

ウ ス ユ ヌ ル フ ム ク ツ ウ
WU SU YU NU LU HU MU KU TU U

IEI

ISO KAMI SHRINE 47 SOUNDS

SE	LI	ME	WA	NE	YA	HI
WE	HE	KA	NU	SI	KO	HU
HO	TE	U	SO	KI	TO	MI
LE	NO	O	WO	LU	MO	YO
KE	MA	E	TA	YU	TI	I
	SU	NI	HA	WI	LO	MU
	A	SA	KU	TU	LA	NA

32 CHILD SOUNDS

NA	LE	HA	SE	KU	YA	TA
KO	NO	NU	HO	MU	YU	TO
	NE	LA	HE	SU	YE	YO
	KA	SA	HU	LU	KE	TU
	MA	LO	MO	SO	ME	TE

SOUND CARD INSTRUCTIONS

To practice sounds:

Sounds may be held for an entire breath, or done quickly. Try different ways, to see which ones work for your study at any given time.

The first prayer [sound card page two], the Amatu Nolito, is read from left to right, as in English. The indicated stops (squares) are places to breathe. This prayer is done once.

Next, go to the back [page four] of the card. The top prayer is the Iso Kami Shrine prayer. It is pronounced from top to bottom, starting at the right, as in ***HI, HU, MI, YO***... This prayer is done three times.

The 32 Child Sounds are also practiced top to bottom, beginning at the right, as in ***TA, TO, YO, TU, TE***... Practice this order three times.

The final practice is on page three. Each order of civilization is practiced separately. They go from top to bottom, starting at the right, *A, I, U, E, O*..., then right to left, starting at the top, *A, KA, SA, TA, NA*...

The orders may also be short-cut: *A, I, U, E, O, WA, WI, WU, WE, WO* each set of five repeated several times, with one final kiai of *Wn!* Then, *A, O, U, E, I, WA, WO, WU, WE, WI,* each set several times, followed by *An!* And finally, *A, I, E, O, U, WA, WI, WE, WO, WU,* each set several times, finished with *IEI!*

The Amatu Futonolito order, the order of the next civilization's consciousness, should also be practiced in its entirety, and can be done with or without the other two. It can be practiced slowly, or fast, once or a hundred times, *A, I, E, O, U*..., then *A, TA, KA, MA, HA, LA*... Breaths, if taken, may be at the end of a line, or after *E* sounds, and *H* sounds. At the end of the *U* line of sounds, pronounce the kiai *IEI!* strongly from your tanden.

OTHER BOOKS BY

MIKOTO MASAHILO NAKAZONO

Current Titles
My Past Way of Budo and other Essays. 1978
Inochi - The Book of Life. 1984
The Source of the Present Civilization. 1994
The Source of the Old and New Testaments. 2007

Out of Print
Messiah's Return. 1972
Kototama. 1976
Ancient World History - Translations from the Takeuti Documents. 1977

Please direct correspondence to:
info@kototamabooks.com
www.kototamabooks.com

For editions in French and Spanish, please contact:
info@kototamabooks.com
www.kototamabooks.com

For editions available in German, please contact:
info@pkp-verlag.de
www.pkp-verlag.de

www.ingramcontent.com/pod-product-compliance
Lightning Source LLC
Chambersburg PA
CBHW070812280326
41934CB00012B/3171

* 9 7 8 0 9 7 1 6 6 7 4 3 3 *